BALANCED BITES

A Recipe Guide for Blood Sugar Monitoring and Wellness.

By

Dr. Howard D. Plante

Copyright © by Dr. Howard D. Plante

2023. All rights reserved.

Before this document is duplicated or reproduced in any manner, the publisher's consent must be gained. Therefore, the contents within can neither be stored electronically, transferred, nor kept in a database. Neither in Part nor full can the document be copied, scanned, faxed, or retained without approval from the publisher or creator.

TABLE OF CONTENT

SUMMARY 4

INTRODUCTION 6

BLOOD SUGAR BASICS............................... 9

BREAKFAST RECIPES.............................. 17

LUNCH AND DINNER RECIPES 23

SNACKS AND APPETIZERS 30

SWEET TREATS 36

MEAL PLANNING AND PREPARATION TIPS 42

CONCLUSION... 48

SUMMARY

Balanced Bites: A Recipe Guide for Blood Sugar Monitoring and Wellness is a comprehensive eBook that balances blood sugar levels for optimal health and wellness. This guide offers delicious and nutrient-rich recipes, meal planning advice, and blood sugar management strategies.

The eBook introduces blood sugar balance and its significant health effects. You'll learn about blood sugar science, common imbalances, and how blood sugar affects your health.

The eBook provides practical advice on blood sugar monitoring and interpretation. You'll learn to make diet and lifestyle choices to control blood sugar. The eBook also emphasizes meal planning and preparation for blood sugar control.

Recipes make the eBook. Each formula promotes healthy blood sugar levels, from breakfast to lunch and dinner to snacks, appetizers, and sweets. Step-by-step instructions make it easy to cook these dishes.

The eBook includes recipes, tips for adapting recipes, and time-saving meal prep strategies. Creating a blood sugar-friendly meal plan and grocery shopping will help you make mindful choices and adopt a balanced bites lifestyle.

The eBook ends with a motivational message and resources to support this lifestyle. Balanced Bites provides the knowledge, inspiration, and recipes you need to achieve blood sugar balance and long-term wellness.

Balanced Bites: A Recipe Guide for Blood Sugar Monitoring and Wellness can change your life.

INTRODUCTION

Thank you for visiting Balanced Bites: A Recipe Guide for Blood Sugar Monitoring and Wellness!

Maintaining a healthy lifestyle in today's fast-paced environment might sometimes feel daunting. We recognize the significance of balancing eating good foods with caring for our bodies. That's why we wrote this eBook: to give you a thorough recipe guide that tantalizes your taste sensations and helps your general health and well-being.

Understanding the significance of blood sugar balance in general health is critical. The foods we eat directly impact our blood sugar levels, affecting our energy levels, weight management, mood stability, and long-term health effects. When our blood sugar levels are consistent, we have better attention, more energy throughout the day, and overall vitality.

You'll learn the practical skills you need from this eBook to monitor and maintain healthy blood sugar levels. Optimal wellness is within your grasp, and our meticulously designed recipes will demonstrate how delicious and fun blood sugar-friendly meals can be.

We've curated a range of nutritious and delicious dishes so you never have to sacrifice flavor while prioritizing your health.

This eBook has a variety of delicious breakfasts, filling lunch and supper options, tempting snacks and appetizers, guilt-free sweet treats, and refreshing beverages. Each recipe has been carefully developed with blood sugar balance principles in mind, using healthful ingredients and sensible portion sizes.

This eBook will not only present you with a wide variety of recipe alternatives, but it also walks you through generating individualized meal plans and provide practical recommendations for grocery shopping and meal preparation. We help you manage your health by incorporating balanced bits into your daily life.

Prepare to embark on a delectable gastronomic trip in which each bite is meticulously crafted to feed your body and boost your overall well-being.

Allow Balanced Bites: A Recipe Guide for Blood Sugar Monitoring and Wellness to be your guide to reaching optimal wellness one delicious and balanced meal at a time.

Will you change eat and feel? Let's look at the tremendous potential of balanced bites for a healthier, happier you!

BLOOD SUGAR BASICS

The Scientific Rationale behind the Measurement of Blood Sugar

Investigating the science that underlies the need to maintain a healthy blood sugar balance is necessary to achieve this goal. Blood sugar, also known as glucose, is an essential component of our bodies since it is an energy source. When we eat carbs, our bodies convert those foods into glucose, which travels via our circulatory system. This glucose is subsequently sent to our cells, serving as a source of fuel for various cellular processes.

Common factors contributing to imbalances in blood sugar

Unfortunately, how we live in the current era frequently contributes to blood sugar abnormalities.

Blood sugar levels can surge and plummet due to sedentary habits, wrong eating patterns, and heavy consumption of refined sweets and processed foods.

In addition, the delicate balance of the body's blood sugar management can be thrown off by external variables such as stress, insufficient sleep, and certain medical diseases.

The Connection between Glucose Levels in the Blood and Overall Health

Managing our energy levels throughout the day is just one of the many benefits of maintaining normal blood sugar levels; it also significantly impacts our bodies' health as a whole. Blood sugar levels that remain elevated for an extended period are associated with an increased likelihood of acquiring chronic disorders such as type 2 diabetes, cardiovascular diseases, and obesity.

On the other side, having blood sugar levels that fluctuate frequently might lead to feelings of weariness, irritability, and difficulty concentrating.

We may begin to comprehend the relevance of adopting a lifestyle that supports balanced blood sugar levels if we understand the connection between blood sugar and overall health.

This understanding can be gained by knowing the link between blood sugar and overall health. It is not just about avoiding disease but also about achieving thriving health, consistent vitality, and enhanced well-being oneself.

How to Keep an Eye on and Make Sense of, Your Blood Sugar Readings

Your blood sugar level should be monitored to ensure that you are in the best possible health.

Finger stick glucometers and continuous glucose monitoring devices are only two examples of the many approaches that can be utilized in determining the sugar level in one's blood.

By monitoring your blood sugar levels regularly, you can trace the patterns of your blood sugar levels, recognize any potential triggers, and make more informed decisions about the foods you eat.

Readings of your blood sugar require more than just knowing the numbers to interpret them correctly. It entails grasping the influence that various diets, stress levels, physical exercise, and other aspects of your lifestyle have on your blood sugar levels. With this newfound information at your disposal, you can make alterations to your diet and lifestyle to help you achieve your general health and well-being objectives.

In the following chapters of this e-book, we will discuss valuable tactics, mouthwatering recipes, and helpful hints for meal planning that can assist you in achieving and sustaining balanced levels of blood sugar.

Remember that striking a healthy balance is essential to realizing your best potential for health and wellness.

Let's keep moving forward on our quest to find more well-rounded bites and, in the process, learn how just a few minor tweaks can significantly benefit your blood sugar and overall health.

BUILDING A BALANCED PLATE

It is vital to plan meals in such a way that they supply a harmonic blend of nutrients to achieve and maintain balanced levels of blood sugar. Within the context of this chapter, "building a balanced plate" refers to ensuring that each meal contributes to achieving one's blood sugar goals and general wellness.

The Elements That Make Up a Meal That Is Beneficial to One's Blood Sugar

A meal is considered "blood sugar friendly" if it contains a balance of macronutrients—carbohydrates, proteins, and fats—that, when consumed together, help maintain stable blood sugar levels. In this section, we will talk about the appropriate amounts and sources of different macronutrients, focusing on their role in maintaining a healthy glucose level in your blood.

Essential Nutrients for Maintaining a Healthy Blood Sugar Level and Overall Wellness

Consuming particular foods can profoundly affect blood sugar and overall health. In this section, we will investigate the role of certain essential nutrients, such as fiber, healthy fats, and lean proteins, in maintaining stable blood sugar levels. You can achieve your wellness objectives more effectively and control your blood sugar by including some of these nutrient powerhouses in your meals.

Techniques for Keeping Track of Your Portions and Planning Your Meals

Regarding keeping blood sugar levels in check, portion control is crucial. In this part of our recipe, we will offer some helpful advice and strategies for controlling portion sizes, which will assist you in achieving a healthy balance on your plate.

In addition, we will discuss the significance of meal planning and offer suggestions on making the process more manageable to facilitate the availability of nutritious and well-balanced meals during the week.

Making Wise Food Choices to Maintain a Normal Blood Sugar Level

Not all foods are created equal regarding how they affect blood sugar levels. We will present a thorough list of foods that are good for maintaining a healthy blood sugar level and discuss the glycemic index and glycemic load of these items. You can make more educated decisions and plan meals more conducive to reaching your overall blood sugar objectives if you know how various foods affect blood sugar.

As we continue reading this e-book, you will come across various dishes for breakfast, lunch, supper, snacks, and desserts that conform to the principles of making a balanced plate. Each recipe has been thoughtfully developed to include the appropriate proportions of nutrients, which will assist you in achieving and sustaining stable blood sugar levels while allowing you to enjoy a wide variety of delectable flavors.

You will be equipped with the resources necessary to produce well-rounded, blood sugar-friendly meals supporting your journey toward optimal wellness if you implement the knowledge obtained in this chapter and utilize the recipes in the following sections.

Next, let's go on to Chapter 4 and investigate the tasty breakfast recipes waiting for you there.

Always remember that taking balanced bites is the key to a balanced life.

BREAKFAST RECIPES

These nutritional and blood sugar-friendly breakfast recipes are the perfect way to get your day off to a good start. These recipes are intended to give a healthy balance of the three types of macronutrients, which will help you get your metabolism going in the morning and maintain a consistent blood sugar level throughout the day. Make your choice from among the following delicious and stimulating breakfast options by carefully following the step-by-step instructions:

1. **Energizing Morning Smoothie**

Ingredients:

1 ripe banana

1 cup spinach

½ cup unsweetened almond milk

1 tablespoon almond butter

1 tablespoon chia seeds

½ teaspoon cinnamon

Ice cubes (optional)

Instructions:

➢ After peeling it, throw the banana in a blender and continue.

➢ The blender should add the following ingredients: spinach, almond milk, almond butter, chia seeds, and cinnamon.

➢ If you prefer your smoothie on the cooler side, feel free to stir in a few ice cubes.

➢ Combine all of the ingredients in a blender until they are silky smooth.

➢ After pouring the smoothie into a glass, you may savor this energizing and nutrient-dense beverage for breakfast.

2. Protein-Packed Veggie Omelet

Ingredients:

3 large eggs

¼ cup diced bell peppers

¼ cup chopped spinach

2 tablespoons diced onions

2 tablespoons grated low-fat cheddar cheese

Salt and pepper to taste

Cooking spray or a small amount of olive oil

➤ In a bowl, beat the eggs with a whisk until thoroughly combined. Add little salt and pepper before serving.

➤ Cooking spray or very little olive oil can give a non-stick skillet a light coating before preheating it in the oven.

➤ The bell peppers, spinach, and onions should all be cut and diced before being added to the skillet. Sauté until the vegetables are soft.

➤ After the eggs have been beaten, pour them over the vegetables that have been sautéed and make sure they are distributed equally.

➤ Please refrain from stirring the omelet for the next few minutes while it is cooking so that the edges can begin to solidify.

➤ One-half of the omelet should have shredded cheddar cheese sprinkled over it in an equal layer.

➤ The remaining half of the omelet should be gently folded over the cheese side using a spatula.

➤ Continue cooking for one more minute or until the cheese melts and the omelet is finished, whichever comes first.

➢ Place the omelet on a dish and serve it warm for a breakfast that is high in protein and has a variety of vegetables. Do this to get your day off to a good start.

3. Whole Grain Banana Pancakes

Ingredients:

1 cup whole wheat flour

1 tablespoon honey or maple syrup

1 teaspoon baking powder

¼ teaspoon salt

1 ripe banana, mashed

1 cup unsweetened almond milk

1 teaspoon vanilla extract

Cooking spray or a small amount of butter for greasing the pan

Instructions:

- Put the honey or maple syrup, baking powder, and salt into a mixing bowl. Add the whole wheat flour and stir to blend.

- The ripe banana should be mashed in a separate bowl until completely smooth. Combine the mashed banana with the almond milk and vanilla essence until well combined.

- After pouring the banana mixture into the dry ingredients, whisk everything together until it is completely incorporated. Take care to keep the elements the same.

- Cooking spray or a tiny amount of butter can lightly lubricate a non-stick skillet or griddle before placing it on a pan or griddle over medium heat.

- Pour the pancake batter onto the griddle using a measuring cup with a capacity of a quarter of a cup to create circular pancakes.

- When you see bubbles beginning to develop on the surface of the pancakes, it's time to flip them over and continue cooking for another minute or until golden brown.

> Proceed with the process with the remaining batter, adjusting the amount of cooking spray or butter you use according to your needs.

> Warm the whole grain banana pancakes and pour them with honey or fresh fruit, if you like those sweeter than they already are, before serving them.

You can cook a breakfast that will provide you with the nutrients and satisfaction you need to go through the day if you follow these step-by-step directions. These recipes can help you maintain healthy blood sugar levels while providing the vitality and food you require for a successful morning. Have fun with your well-balanced snacks, and prepare for the day's challenges!

LUNCH AND DINNER RECIPES

Treat yourself to these delicious lunch and dinner recipes that help you achieve your blood sugar objectives. These dishes will keep you satiated and energized throughout the day. To make these delightful dishes, follow the step-by-step instructions that are listed below:

1. Grilled Chicken and Quinoa Salad

Ingredients:

1 boneless, skinless chicken breast

½ cup cooked quinoa

2 cups mixed salad greens

½ cup cherry tomatoes, halved

¼ cup sliced cucumbers

2 tablespoons diced red onions

2 tablespoons feta cheese, crumbled

2 tablespoons extra virgin olive oil

1 tablespoon lemon juice

Salt and pepper to taste

Instructions:

1. Prepare a grill or pan by heating it to a medium-high temperature.

2. The chicken breast needs to be seasoned with salt and pepper.

3. Grill the chicken until it reaches 165°F (74°C) on each side. Cool down.

4. Mix cooked quinoa, mixed salad greens, cherry tomatoes, cucumbers, and red onions in a large bowl.

5. In a small bowl, combine the extra virgin olive oil, lemon juice, salt, and pepper to make the dressing.

6. Cut the chicken breast into thin pieces after grilling.

7. Add feta cheese and chicken strips to the salad.

8. Drizzle the dressing on the salad and stir.

9. Serve the grilled chicken and quinoa salad for a healthy supper.

2. Roasted Salmon with Lemon and Asparagus

Ingredients:

2 salmon fillets
1 bunch asparagus, trimmed
1 tablespoon olive oil
1 lemon, sliced
2 cloves garlic, minced
Salt and pepper to taste

Instructions:

1. Start preheating the oven immediately to 400°F (200°C).
2. Put the salmon pieces on a baking sheet lined with parchment paper.
3. Place the fish and the trimmed asparagus on a baking sheet.
4. Drizzle olive oil over the salmon and asparagus, then equally sprinkle minced garlic, salt, and pepper over both.
5. Put lemon pieces on top of the salmon fillets.
6. Roast the salmon in an oven that has been warm for about 12 to 15 min until wholly cooked and comes apart easily with a fork.
7. Take the salmon out of the oven and serve it with lemon and asparagus for a tasty and healthy meal.

3. Turkey and Veggie Stir-Fry

Ingredients:

1 tablespoon olive oil

1 pound ground turkey

1 red bell pepper, sliced

1 zucchini, sliced

1 carrot, sliced

½ cup snap peas

2 cloves garlic, minced

2 tablespoons low-sodium soy sauce

1 tablespoon hoisin sauce

1 teaspoon sesame oil

Sesame seeds for garnish (optional)

Instructions

1. Place the olive oil in a big ring the oil to a boil in a pan or wok at medium temperature.

2. Add the ground turkey and sauté it, chopping it into small pieces as it cooks until it has browned.

3. Add the sliced red bell pepper, zucchini, carrot, snap peas, and minced garlic, and stir to combine.

4. cook for approximately 5 to 6 minutes or until the veggies reach a crisp-tender consistency.

5. Combine the low-sodium soy sauce and hoisin sauce; in a low-sided bowl, combine the olive oil and the soy sauce and whisk together until smooth.

6. Add the sauce to the skillet containing the turkey and vegetable combination, and stir to combine.

7. Give everything a good stir to get a uniform coating, and then continue cooking for another two to three minutes to bring it up to temperature.

8. If you want to add more flavor and appearance, sprinkle on some sesame seeds.

9. As a delicious and healthy choice for lunch or dinner, serve the turkey and vegetable stir-fry to your guests.

4. Lentil and Vegetable Curry

Ingredients:

1 tablespoon olive oil

1 onion, diced

2 cloves garlic, minced

1 tablespoon curry powder

1 teaspoon ground cumin

1 teaspoon ground coriander

1 cup dried lentils, rinsed

1 can (14 ounces) diced tomatoes

2 cups vegetable broth

1 cup chopped vegetables of your choice (e.g., bell peppers, carrots, cauliflower)

Salt and pepper to taste

Fresh cilantro for garnish (optional)

Instructions

1. Prepare the olive oil in a large pot over medium heat.

2. Crush the garlic cloves and add the onion cut to the pot. Cook the onion over medium heat until you can see through it.

3. Stir in the curry, cumin, and coriander powders to bring out the flavours. About a minute is enough time to cook.

4. Add the washed lentils, the cut tomatoes, the vegetable broth, and the chopped vegetables to the pot.

5. If desired, add salt and pepper.

6. Lower the heat and boil the ingredients; cover the pot.

7. Simmer for 25–30 minutes until beans and vegetables are soft.

8. To prevent sticking, stir it frequently; if you need to, add more vegetable broth.

9. You can serve the lentil and vegetable soup with cooked quinoa or brown rice and fresh cilantro on top.

These meals for lunch and dinner are designed to be both satiating and friendly to blood sugar levels, ensuring that you are well-nourished and have plenty of energy throughout the day. Savour the delectable flavours while reaping their beneficial effects on your health.

SNACKS AND APPETIZERS

Treat yourself to these delectable snacks and appetizers that are delicious and beneficial to one's blood sugar. These dishes will fulfil your desires while providing a boost of nutrients.

1. **Crunchy Kale Chips**

Ingredients:

1 bunch kale, stems removed and torn into bite-sized pieces

1 tablespoon olive oil

½ teaspoon salt

Optional seasonings: garlic powder, paprika, or nutritional yeast

Instructions

1. Prepare the oven for 350°F (175 °C).
2. Put the kale leaves that have been torn into a wide basin.
3. The kale should be seasoned with salt, and olive oil should be drizzled.

4. Please give them a good toss to ensure the oil and salt are distributed uniformly across the kale leaves.

5. Sprinkling the chosen seasonings over the kale is optional to add some taste.

6. Use a parchment-lined baking sheet with the kale leaves spread out in a single layer on the sheet.

7. Bake for 10–15 minutes until the edges are golden and crispy.

8. After baking, let the kale chips cool before serving. Kale chips are a tasty, guilt-free snack.

2. Avocado Toast with Tomato and Sprouts

Ingredients:

2 slices whole grain bread, toasted

1 ripe avocado, mashed

½ cup cherry tomatoes, halved

¼ cup sprouts (e.g., alfalfa sprouts or broccoli sprouts)

Salt and pepper to taste

Optional toppings: red pepper flakes or balsamic glaze

Instructions:

1. Spread avocado on toasted bread.

2. Cherry tomatoes and sprouts with avocado.

3. Salt & pepper to taste.

4. Optional: Add red pepper flakes for spice or balsamic glaze for tang.

5. Avocado toast with tomato and sprouts is a healthy snack or appetizer.

3. Spicy Edamame Dip

Ingredients:

1 cup shelled edamame, cooked according to package instructions

2 tablespoons tahini

1 tablespoon fresh lemon juice

1 clove garlic, minced

½ teaspoon ground cumin

½ teaspoon chili powder

¼ teaspoon cayenne pepper (adjust to taste)

Salt to taste

Optional toppings: chopped green onions or sesame seeds

Instructions:

1. Put the edamame that has been cooked, the tahini, the lemon juice, the minced garlic, the ground cumin, the chili powder, the cayenne pepper, and the salt into a food processor.
2. Run the processor until the mixture is silky smooth and creamy, stopping to scrape down the sides as necessary.
3. Taste the dish, then make any necessary adjustments to the spices to suit your tastes.
4. Move the dip to a bowl that will be used for serving.
5. To enhance both the flavor and the appearance of the dish, a garnish of chopped green onions or toasted sesame seeds can be used.
6. Serve spicy edamame dip with sliced vegetables, whole grain crackers, or pita chips for a snack that is both flavorful and high in protein.

4. Zucchini Fritters with Greek Yogurt Sauce

Ingredients:

2 medium zucchini, grated
1 teaspoon salt
1 egg, beaten

¼ cup whole wheat flour
2 tablespoons grated Parmesan cheese
2 green onions, finely chopped
1 clove garlic, minced
¼ teaspoon black pepper
2 tablespoons olive oil (for frying)
Greek yogurt sauce for dipping

Instructions:

1. After grating the zucchini, place it in a sieve and season it with salt. Allow it to rest for about ten minutes so that the excess moisture may be released.

2. Squeeze the zucchini with a clean dish towel or several paper towels to remove any extra liquid that may have accumulated.

3. Grated zucchini, an egg that has been beaten, whole wheat flour, grated Parmesan cheese, chopped green onions, minced garlic, and black pepper should be mixed together in a big basin. Combine all of the components by thoroughly combining the ingredients.

4. Prepare olive oil in a pan over medium heat.

5. Take roughly 2 teaspoons of the zucchini mixture and form it into a ball before flattening it into the shape of a fritter. Repeat the same with the remaining portion of the mixture, taking care not to crowd the pan too much.

6. Fry the fritters for approximately three to four minutes on each side, or until they are crisp and golden brown.

7. Put the fried fritters on a platter that has been coated with paper towels so that any excess oil may be absorbed.

8. To use as a dipping sauce, the zucchini fritters should be served alongside a serving of Greek yogurt. These savory fritters are perfect for a snack or an appetizer since they are both nutritious and tasty.

These snacks and appetizers will delight your taste buds while also helping you meet your blood sugar goals. As you go about your day, treat yourself to a few of these savory morsels that are also loaded with nutrients.

SWEET TREATS

Enjoy these delicious sweets without worrying about their effect on your blood sugar levels. The ingredients and flavors in these dishes are both healthy and delightful. To make these delicious treats, just follow the steps outlined below.

1. **Berry Parfait with Greek Yogurt**

Ingredients:

1 cup Greek yogurt

½ cup mixed berries (strawberries, blueberries, raspberries)

¼ cup granola

1 tablespoon honey (optional)

Fresh mint leaves for garnish (optional)

Instructions:

1. Spread a quarter of the Greek yogurt on the bottom of a glass or dish.
2. Sprinkle a quarter of the mixed berries over the yogurt
3. Cover the berries with half of the granola.

4. Add the rest of the Greek yogurt, berries, and granola, and repeat the layering process.

5. If you like honey, you can drizzle some on top.

6. Use mint leaves as a garnish for a burst of brightness.

7. The berry parfait is a healthy and refreshing dessert option.

2. Chocolate Avocado Mousse

Ingredients:

2 ripe avocados

¼ cup unsweetened cocoa powder

¼ cup pure maple syrup or honey

¼ cup almond milk or any non-dairy milk

1 teaspoon vanilla extract

Pinch of salt

Optional toppings: sliced strawberries or shaved dark chocolate.

Instructions:

1. Blend or process ripe avocados, unsweetened chocolate powder, maple syrup or honey, almond milk, vanilla extract, and salt.

2. Blend until creamy, scraping the sides.

3. Taste and adjust the sweetness.

4. Serve chocolate avocado mousse in ramekins.

5. Refrigerate for 30 minutes.

6. Add extravagance with sliced strawberries or shaved dark chocolate.

7. Chocolate avocado mousse is a delicious, healthy chocolate treat.

3. Almond Flour Blueberry Muffins

Ingredients:

2 cups almond flour

½ teaspoon baking soda

¼ teaspoon salt

3 tablespoons coconut oil, melted

¼ cup pure maple syrup or honey

3 large eggs

1 teaspoon vanilla extract

1 cup fresh blueberries.

Instructions:

1. Bake at 350°F (175°C). Paper-line a muffin tray.
2. Whisk almond flour, baking soda, and salt in a large bowl.
3. Whisk melted coconut oil, maple syrup or honey, eggs, and vanilla extract in a separate basin.
4. Put the wet ingredients in the dry bowl. Mix thoroughly.
5. Add fresh blueberries.
6. Put three-quarters of a cup of batter into each muffin tin.
7. A toothpick put into a muffin should come clean after 20–25 minutes.
8. After baking, let the muffins rest before moving them to a wire rack to cool.
9. Almond-flour blueberry muffins are a healthy dessert.

4. Coconut Energy Bites

Ingredients:

1 cup shredded unsweetened coconut

½ cup almond flour

¼ cup pure maple syrup or honey

2 tablespoons coconut oil, melted

1 teaspoon vanilla extract

Pinch of salt

Optional add-ins: chopped nuts, dried fruits, or chocolate chips

Instructions:

1. Mix almond flour and unsweetened coconut in a large bowl.
2. Whisk maple syrup or honey, melted coconut oil, vanilla extract, and salt in another bowl.
3. Put the wet ingredients in the dry bowl. Blend well.
4. Optional: Add chopped nuts, dried fruit, or chocolate chips.
5. Form bite-sized balls with your hands.
6. Coconut energy bites on a parchment-lined baking sheet.
7. Refrigerate for 30 minutes to set.

8. Energy bites can be refrigerated for a week in an airtight container.

9. Coconut energy bites are a healthy, portable snack.

These sugar-free treats will satisfy your sweet tooth. These healthy and delicious recipes will satisfy your sweet tooth.

MEAL PLANNING AND PREPARATION TIPS

Planning and preparing meals well is essential to keep a good blood sugar diet and be as healthy as possible. Follow these step-by-step instructions to make it easy to plan and cook your balanced bites:

1. Making a Meal Plan That's Good for Your Blood Sugar

Step 1:

Know what you want and why.

Determine your dietary requirements, considering your goals for managing your blood sugar and overall health.

Consider personal tastes, dietary restrictions, or food allergies when planning meals.

Step 2: Plan healthy meals

Eat lean proteins, whole grains, healthy fats, and many fruits and vegetables.

Aim for a balance of macronutrients (carbohydrates, proteins, and fats) to help keep your blood sugar stable.

Consider portion sizes to ensure you get enough nutrients without overeating.

Step 3: Have meals and snacks at different times of the day

Plan for three main meals and two to three snacks daily to keep your blood sugar levels steady and stop you from getting too hungry.

Schedule your meals and snacks regularly to keep your energy levels steady and your blood sugar from going up and down too much.

2. Shopping for Food to Make Balanced Bites

First, make a list.

Review your meal plan and complete a grocery list based on your balanced bites.

Include essential items that should always be in the pantry and any special items your recipes call for.

Step 2: Choose good ingredients.

Focus on fresh and whole foods, such as fruits, vegetables, lean proteins, whole grains, and healthy fats.

Choose organic produce from your area or in a season when you can.

Read food labels to avoid added sugars, artificial ingredients, and processed foods that can throw off the blood sugar balance.

Step 3: Plan your shopping.

To avoid buying unnecessary items and ensure you have everything for planned meals, stick to your grocery list.

Think about shopping outside the grocery store, where most fresh produce, meat, and dairy products are kept.

You can save time and be more convenient by ordering groceries online or delivering them.

3. Ways to save time on meal prep

Step 1: Plan your preparation day.

Schedule weekly meal prep.

Choose a day when you have more free time, like the weekend or the evening, to focus on making your meals and dividing them up.

Step 2: Cook meals in bulk and divide them up.

Cook more proteins, grains, and roasted vegetables at once to use them for more than one meal during the week.

Divide the cooked parts into individual portions or meal containers to make them easy and quick to assemble.

Step 3: Cut and prepare the food ahead of time

To save time when making a meal, wash, chop, and prepare fruits, vegetables, and herbs ahead of time.

Store ingredients that have already been cut in airtight containers or bags in the fridge to keep them fresh.

4. Making Recipes Work for You

Step 1: Know what goes into a recipe.

Learn about the main parts of a recipe, like proteins, carbohydrates, and fats.

Find out if any ingredients must be changed or replaced to help you reach your blood sugar goals.

Step 2: Make Smart Ingredient Swaps

Whole grains, like brown rice or quinoa, should be used instead of refined grains.

Instead of refined sugar, use natural sweeteners like honey or pure maple syrup.

Instead of frying, choose cooking methods that are better for you, such as baking, grilling, or steaming.

Step 3: Check the sizes of the servings

To meet your blood sugar management goals, adjust your portion sizes.

Be aware of ingredients high in carbohydrates and ensure they are balanced with enough protein and healthy fats.

Using these tips for planning and making meals, you can keep your blood sugar level and overall health at their best. Enjoy the ease of organized meal plans, efficient grocery shopping, and time-saving ways to prepare meals to help you live a healthier life.

CONCLUSION

With Balanced Bites: A Recipe Guide for Blood Sugar Monitoring and Wellness, you've taken the first step toward healthy eating and good blood sugar. By putting the ideas and recipes in this eBook into practice, you are taking steps to improve your health and well-being.

Taking on the Balanced Bites way of life

You have learned a lot from this eBook about how vital blood sugar balance is and how it can be good for your health. By living the Balanced Bites way of life, you put nutrient-dense foods first, plan your meals carefully, and make choices that help you reach your blood sugar goals.

Keeping blood sugar in check is essential for long-term health.

Remember that balancing your blood sugar and keeping it that way is an ongoing process. It takes consistency, awareness of yourself, and intelligent choices about the foods you eat. You can improve your overall health and maximize your wellness by watching how much you eat, choosing whole, unprocessed foods, and monitoring your blood sugar levels.

Remember that balancing your blood sugar is an ongoing process that requires patience, self-care, and a commitment to feeding your body healthy, well-balanced meals. The recipes and tips in this eBook are meant to get you started on this path and give you the power to keep going.

I hope you have success, good health, and a life full of well-balanced bites!

www.ingramcontent.com/pod-product-compliance
Lightning Source LLC
Chambersburg PA
CBHW061531250726

48657CB00005B/2170